Rebuilding a Broken Body for a Youthful Tomorrow

I0102326

Sam Morishima

with Michael Yanuck MD PhD

DEDICATION

**For Shiatsu master, Stephen Tamaribuchi,
and Michael Yanuck MD PhD**

.

CONTENTS

Disclaimer.

This is a story of rebuilding my body and how I approached it. I cannot say it would apply to others, like saying one size fits all. It only works if you are my size. If so, then maybe my journey is a premonition to take note. Challenge what I say and question all ideas derived from my words. I do not endorse nor recommend any of the ideas and methods in this writing. Nothing in this writing is of a nature of a scientific study or body of scientific work. Again, it is my views of a journey to become physically and mentally better. Here is my anecdotal approach to my life's situation to rebuild my broken body.

ACKNOWLEDGEMENTS

I would first like to thank Shiatsu master, Stephen Tamaribuchi, without whom I would not have found the way to improve my body through bio-mechanics. He has not only shown me how critical bio-mechanics are to an efficient, balanced, stronger and skilled dynamic body, but has re-aligned my body many times from past injuries and still many more times from injuries when I pushed myself beyond my limitations. His persistent scolding's when I did things improperly (and yet not giving up on me) have given me a quality of life, filled with activities I thought had passed me by. Most if not all the bio-mechanical exercises and concepts in this writing originated from his work and development in this area.

The second acknowledgement goes to Michael Yanuck MD PhD who like me has not given up on improving his body, discovering it keeps getting better. Discussing our approaches after roller skating at a nearby restaurant (until they usually had to kick us out, so they could close) created an opportunity to mesh our separate styles: My bio-mechanical approach, and his use of both standard medical knowledge and bioenergy, combined with awareness of body, feel and biosense to fully rebuild a body in a coherent way.

Both Stephen Tamaribuchi and Dr. Yanuck helped me understand a fuller picture of the human body as pertains to the awareness of the use of bio-mechanics, medical knowledge and bioenergy to heal and rebuild my body, so that I could continue to grow, with activities (both physical and mental) in a natural, healthy manner, even at an age when most people with injury don't realize the possibilities that still exist to grow and rebuild.

PROLOGUE

Even though I perform what many believe are tricky, difficult and dangerous maneuvers on skates, skis and other riding sports, they are for me normal movements that are part of my being. They don't feel dangerous or tricky or difficult, but natural. The feeling of body coordination is harmonic and rhythmic, and my body seems to just meld with the movement. However, early on as I was developing them, they were risky and harmful, especially under the light of my illness and acquired injuries, pushing myself, thinking that was helping. This is my journey to develop the ability to do these things through rebuilding my broken body under the damaging effects of illnesses and injuries I acquired.

Motivation to achieve higher performance levels was my guiding star, navigating my process of rebuilding my body. In attempting to become successful at each level of achievement, I learned how to improve my body and deal with setbacks. Wandering in the wrong direction taught me to recognize signs to avoid and cease further ruinous actions. It was important to distinguish pain that would damage versus the feeling of pain that is part of the process of rebuilding (such as soreness vs acute sharp pain that meant serious injurious mechanics at play). Soreness was a variable sign indicating that I'd done enough and it was time for a rest; versus when continuing on would result in compensation of other non-optimized biomechanics. Further pushing on meant installment of poor limiting mechanical habits with restraints on performance improvement.

Injuries caused by my ignorance might one day need serious interventions such as surgery. However, my guiding star has been able to pierce through the heavy clouds and fog of fright and despair as I continued to work on my body, experimenting with alignment, bio-mechanics and sensitivity to biosense. However, with that said, I reserve the right to say 'only time will tell.' For now, my body appears to be accommodating my ability to keep improving.

Life is full of risks and sometimes I feel the secret to life is to be able to cope with setbacks and catastrophes. Doing better at the things I like to 'play' such as skiing, snowboarding, skating, surfing, etc. better prepares me to face, cope and overcome the catastrophes in my life.

My stubborn belief I can do better at play is rooted in developing solid fundamentals of skeletal posturing in a neutral alignment that maximizes muscle recruitment providing strong leverage in movements and balance, and sensing them through Bio-sense.

I believe strongly in this fundamental. For when I lose my strong athletic posture of neutral alignment, I instantly lose balance and collapse like when cutting the strings that hold up a marinate puppet. My illness and past injuries have narrowed my tolerance to do things. I am greatly sensitive to the weakening effects of poor athletic posture. Strong bio-mechanics gives me the capabilities to be balanced, stable, stronger, more agile, with greater range of motion, and most importantly, allows me to keep on improving in activities I love to do.

Understanding my tolerance was understanding my limitations and working within them. In time I knew I would broaden my tolerance and extend the boundaries to do things better. Having solid fundamental of good bio-mechanics with a neutral body alignment created proper skills and techniques for sports. With continued practice, using skating and skiing to engrain habits of strong alignment and use of proper biomechanics into my skills and techniques, I was able to drive my sense and alignment posture deep into my movements, expanding my boundaries to reach my limitations. So much so that when I first began roller skating at age 55 to rehabilitate my first knee injury, the following next two years I fell 6 to 10 times during each 2-hour skating session. At first, each fall would startle the other skaters. After a few weeks of me annoying the other skaters by falling (but getting back up), they'd just tell new skaters not to worry about me, saying, "Sam falls all the time."

Now, at over 65, I do complicated moves on skates, and fall only rarely. Improving and growing in my ability to skate, ski, snowboard and many other activities (having younger athletes following my lead in skill and technique development) is an accomplishment I believe was only achieved by my pursuant journey to rebuild my body. I continue to literally skate along the edge of my boundaries of performance by stepping over that boundary line until I am comfortable being over the border, expanding my limitation of tolerance, and being an immigrant in a higher performance level until I am fully assimilated provides me the foundation to migrate to the next higher level.

Strengthening my fundamentals of biomechanics and bio-sense at each level allowed me to push the envelope into the next level by allowing me to develop the skills and techniques to push further.

1 OLD AND INJURED WITH A PASSION TO BE BETTER

At an age of 46 I became ill, so that I had to quit work to focus on healing myself and rebuilding my damaged body. Now at 65 my journey of rebuilding has gone through five different stages. These five stages are determined by injury and an approach to recovery. Each is a journey into understanding how my body deals with detrimental conditions to emerge having grown and expanded in ability, skill and technique. Through my love of activities, I am wiser at understanding my body and mind under this fragile ceiling of health.

Stage 1. Hormonal tragedy and regaining strength and countering lethargy

Stage 2. Left knee injury and an initial biomechanical approach to therapy

Stage3. Right knee injury and a deeper understanding of biomechanical approach to therapy

Stage 4. Overconfidence and reinjury, combining the incorporation of bioenergy awareness and better directed biomechanical approaches to therapy.

Stage 5. Anticipating future prevention

My journey of maximizing and working at becoming healthier, stronger, performing better and staying mentally alert is mingled with the struggle of maintaining my passion for living as an individual and in family life. This struggle has been wrought with a constant vigilance, and working out the optimal way of navigating my awareness of detrimental body changes from my overriding hormonal illness, while pushing my body to be athletically better against factors associated with age. In this constant battle to do more and be better is my love for sports such as ski, snowboard, roller skate, surf, wake board, etc. I discovered that to be young at old age required moving effortlessly with smoothness, stability and skill. I have been surprised at my ability to continue to improve at these sports. It is a thrill when kids and teens come up to me and want to do the things I do and in the way I do them. They are shocked when I answer their question of my age by telling them I'm 65, old enough to be their grandparent. I hope that this writing may help you find youthful vigor that gives you joy and makes you feel alive as you mature into old age.

Dr. Yanuck: As compared to the traumatic experiences I described, bad posture resulting in poor body mechanics don't really represent direct trauma to the body. Rather, bad posture typically comes about because of the day-to-day trauma entailed in poor body use...

2 HOW I GOT HERE

Loving one's job was detrimental to my health. For brevity sake, it happened at 4 AM in my office in California, while working on the business proposal to open up a new country for the company's product. Staying up all night after returning from a demanding tour of countries and a 13-hour flight from Asia, I was expanding my territory of responsibilities in LAMPAC (an acronym for Latin America and Pacific Rim). The flight included Taiwan, Japan, S. Korea, China, Australia and New Zealand (Thank God on this leg I didn't have to stop in Mexico, Brazil or Columbia). My job was to open up and manage the development of new businesses in these countries. It was pretty much left up to me to determine the feasibility of developing new markets, establishing distribution channels, and forming the business and customer infrastructure until the country was established enough to be incorporated and blended into the company structure (typically when the annual product sales are close to $100 million and our product is a market leader in the country, usually in a three-to-five year time frame). In the meantime it was my child and my responsibility to make it happen.

Completing a multilayered forecast spreadsheet for a new country candidate, I thought I had justified another all-night's worth of work. Then, suddenly, I heard a snap. That snap came from my brain. It was clear and distinct, but (in the moment) I gave it no mind – hoping it was nothing. But that marked the beginning of my physical and mental decline. A month later I was a mess: lethargic, unable to think clearly, my strength drained, falling asleep in the middle of meetings. Doctors found that my brain's hypothalamus had somehow changed, and releasing factors were not functioning properly.

One major effect was extremely low testosterone levels. For males we depend on testosterone for muscle tone, bone density, and energy for both physical and mental activities. Supplemental testosterone added some relief, but still felt short of where I'd been in strength and overall wellbeing. This condition was more complicated than just low testosterone.

For more see Appendix A "Science and Slopes," an article about Sam Morishima "a globe-hopping workaholic quits his dizzying schedule and finds a happy marriage between his youthful passion and his penchant for science."

Comment Dr. Yanuck: It strikes me that the 'great' thing about Sam's experience (that is, great for us, not for him) is that he effectively became an 'old man' overnight! In this way he was immediately thrust in a position that he had to adjust/correct his biomechanics so not to fight his body in any way, because he quite literally didn't have the strength to. He had to work with it on its terms (effectively, in its favorite ways of being used), because it would no longer permit him to simply apply his will and power through to make the body and mind do as he wanted.

3 IMPROVING MY DYNAMIC BALANCE

With my hormones off, my physical and mental health went into disarray. I became physically weak, my mind lethargic, with a lack of energy and will most of the time.

Physically, my muscles atrophied to the point that I easily cramped. I cramped in places I never knew you could cramp. It seemed each day I found a new muscle through this process of cramping, especially during my sleeping hours when I least expected it.

In addition to the cramping, I was losing my coordination and strength. It got so bad that one morning (after placing my left foot on the floor), I immediately collapsed. It wasn't that the leg was paralyzed; it was just weak. It took me almost an hour to try and train the leg to hold up my left side, and I did this by making the left leg mimic the movements of the right leg.

(Comment Dr. Yanuck: All of these places of cramping were likely sites of traumatic injury or inappropriate compensation that had not been completely reconciled for Sam, And likely would have responded to modality is like a schema compression and sequential stimulation at Sam known about these modalities at the time.)

That afternoon I ventured outside to see if I could walk around the park near my house. Carefully flexing and extending the left leg and foot, I clumsily walked, resting every few minutes as I went. All this created an awareness of the biomechanics of walking and the need to execute these movements properly, so to achieve dynamic balance.

In this way the ultimate decision to open my home indoor ski school at age of 47 allowed me to focus both my body and mind on physically and mentally challenging myself, at the same time that I taught students. It was a way to develop my coordination and dynamic balance in a unique sense. I discovered that dynamic balance when walking or running is different than in riding mode (such as skiing, snowboarding and roller skating). Discovering the difference allowed me to take apart the process of body movements for these different types of activities and create approaches to improve on the correct technique. It taught me to understand why people have difficulties adapting to different activities especially when they demand opposite set of rules for technique and skills.

Back to my indoor ski school, by teaching and having to master (well enough) on the revolving ski deck allowed me to develop my body and my mind toward a healthier state that allowed me to rebuild myself. An important aspect of becoming stronger in mind and body is to become a good instructor. Being an instructor requires in-depth study and seeking advice from others who were not only athletic champions but were pragmatic in their development. I acquired knowledge of techniques and transferred them not only into my instructions to students but towards my personal improvement in skiing, snowboarding and other riding sports (roller skating, wake boarding, etc.). In a short time I became very accomplished at them basically because I followed a simple 7 step principle which I took from others and modified to my situation:

1. When I trained, I practiced in a manner that would simulate as close as possible to the real thing. In this case skiing and snowboarding on an Endless Slope which is a revolving carpeted slope (more on Revolving ski decks see Appendix __). This simulated the most technically demanding ski and snowboard situation which is steep and icy.

2. Practice proper technique. Working with students I saw what worked and what didn't; what are fundamentals that made them continue to improve and were lasting. I tried it on myself before I passed it on to my students. I worked together with my students and we grew together, quickly and properly. The two most important aspects to improving pointed to: 1. Proper bio-mechanics in ski and snowboard techniques; and 2. feeling the ride through sensing the body in motion so that proper reactions can be initiated by body perception.

3. Keep the practice sessions short but do them frequently. I found that when trying to develop a new skill, it is easy to overdo it, and since it is new, you have not developed the infrastructure to sustain the skill for a long time. Remember, a new technique usually requires fine motor skills and coordinated timing. So, it is important to keep the time short, so you are doing it properly and not fatigue

your body and begin to go from doing it properly to creating a bad habit. Once a bad habit is incorporated they say it takes 7 times more work to break that bad habit and re-install the proper habit. I found that a short and frequent approach to install good habits is a very practical way to reshape my behavior and improve the way I move so that it would not damage my injuries and allow healing. An example is balancing on one leg just in the morning and evening when I brush my teeth. Doing this every day, not only did my balance and weight shifting on skis improve, but my knees that were damaged became stronger and the feelings of pain and unusual sensitivity diminished within weeks. It is now a habit I do without thinking and it is hard not to balance on one leg and then the next when brushing my teeth.

Of note, the fatigue muscles same alludes to here would have likely been amenable to treatment with modalities like ischemic compression and sequential stimulation, so to facilitate a more functional state and healing.

4. Practice time should be used efficiently with focused intent. Being disciplined in practice while working on an activity is a powerful capability that accelerates proficiency.

5. When practicing, utilize the facility and available tools optimally. The Endless Slope is like a laboratory, allowing optimization by reducing the variables to specific needs. During the period I was healing my knees I used a brace to keep the knee stable but allowed the knee cap to track properly as I flexed the knee. I found that utilizing tools this way is a great aid in helping the healing process. I researched several braces and found that fit, feel and function are key to rebuilding, as they minimized the chance of re-injury and yet allow the joint to articulate, so to maintain muscle tone during the healing period, and minimize stiffness and frozen joints.

6. In each practice session success must be experienced. Dynamic balance in riding is complex and when proper developmental training occurs the student will feel a new sensation that will add to the fundamentals of movement. These improvements are endless as we get better and skills are reinforced in our new self. We see this success in our improved performance, and being able to do something we were previously not able to do before.

7. The last thing is for practice be fun and enjoyable. I can honestly say I have fun every time I ride on the Endless Slope because I love to ski and benefit from it building my body's health. Because I developed proper technique that is bio-mechanically sound, it puts little demand on the body and allows ski and snowboard movements to occur which help exercise and heal injury.

I understand I am fortunate to have an Endless Slope. It has literally changed my life for the better. But this is only the beginning chapter in this new phase of my life. For my illness was still with me and what I did was improve my life within the confines of the range it allowed me to live in. I realized that due to my lack of testosterone, it would be very difficult to regain the powerful strength I once had, and bulking up on muscle would be nearly impossible.

My key personnel personal focus back was how to maximize my ability to do things with a condition that was limiting my strength physically, and mentally leaving me feeling tired. From a mental standpoint, multi-tasking was harder, and what I needed was something that offered a narrow focus. The ski school did that, allowing me to exercise in a fun fashion and focus on helping others.

4 THE LESSON OF IMPROVING UNDER DEBILITATING CONDITIONS

The first thing I realized was know your weakness as much as you can so can anticipate how they will hinder your ability to become better. Then figure out ways to get around them or strengthen them so they will not be an obstacle.

Second is that I will not know everything about all my weaknesses, but I learned I will be living through them as I become stronger uncovering them as they become the eliminating link for further development. As that raise their ugly head the key is to recognize them and create a plan to minimize their affect to resist your improvement. Becoming aware and then diagnosing these impinging weaknesses I had to not only be able to feel their onset as they became engaged, such as in my improvement of greater range of motion that required the use of different muscle groups or maybe demanding greater capabilities of the muscles in play. They first showed up as limiting my technique to accomplish an activity effortlessly. If I kept forcing it, what usually happened was I badly injured myself. It is important to study your current technique and learn about what you are trying to accomplish. This latter would require from me a lot of book reading and research about the kinetics of what I am trying to achieve. The third is to create a plan that would help me develop either of both a change in technique or development of a new technique. The Fourth is to practice and practice to incorporate the techniques. Since this is a work in progress be conscientious that modification and changing of practice is usually necessary...

5 INJURY ON TOP OF INJURY

A caution is that when you feel and perform better you tend to overdo things. Feeling stronger both mentally and physically as well as high improvements in performance made me push the envelope further to see how far I could go. Even thoughts of competing and doing things that very few people are capable of. That is when you try to do something you are not quite ready for. That is when I injured my legs to the point of permanent damage that now restricts my range of performance movement.

First, I tore the Medial Collateral Ligament (MCL) of my left knee. When it seemed the knee was becoming well (though not quite fully recovered) I was teaching on the mountain and practicing a jump. But I landed hard, and my right leg collapsed. Compensating for the not quite healed left knee had most likely resulted in misalignments, and the right knee gave way to the impact, and it turned out I had torn the MCL and meniscus of my right leg.

Laying there not able to move, a sense of fear ran through me. Maybe this was the big injury that would cripple me, I though, and the confusion of what to do next so that I do not worsen the situation.

Attempting to immobilize the right leg, there was a shock of pain and then lack of movement and /or, weakness, swelling, feeling of heat and imaging discoloration of injury site.

Trying to focus through the pain and what ifs of types of damages done, I tried to extract myself from this place and get some appropriate treatment.

Still, laying at the bottom of the jump I was glad no one else was coming. It was the end of the day, and I was pretty much the last person on the hill. After a brief rest I got up on one ski and managed to ski on my left leg to the gondola that took me down the mountain. I remember the ride down as the gondola passed over the mogul fields of Gun Barrel at Heavenly and I wondered, Will I ever go down these bumps again on skis?

These fresh injuries that will likely limit me permanently. How do I know? If I go off balance beyond which would be normal balance for an uninjured person, my legs collapse out from under me.

Fortunately, not long after this injury, I met Stephen Taramibuchi, who introduced me to body mechanics. He helped me understand the importance of Bio-mechanics and skeletal alignment regarding strength and leverage. Under his care he helped align my knees, hips back and neck so that my skeletal frame was properly stacked. He showed me what to do with my hands and feet when sitting, standing, walking, and moving that will maintain good posture and alignment. He provided me with exercises that would allow appropriate patterning of movements that would allow maximal muscle recruitment for strength and leverage.

What I have discovered is the more precise and accurate my alignment, the more stable my dynamic balance, and my legs hold me up. However, if I go beyond that, my legs become jello and my body structure loses all strength and collapses.

My tolerance is very narrow, but as long as I am within it, I can do amazing things. My main practice focus are ways to keep appropriate posture that provides proper alignment, strong leverage and maximal muscle recruitment. From there I can work on agility and toning the muscles. Ability to focus on these basic elements allows me to enjoy activities roller skating, walking with poles, skiing and snowboarding.

I continue to 'push the envelope' (as this is part of my nature) and hence continue to reinjure my body. And by God it feels great to go beyond yesterday's mark...

6 WE TEND TO DO THINGS THAT CAUSE THE THING WE WANT TO AVOID

On a recent visit to Stephen Tamaribuchi, he pointed out how my pelvis was rolling under me, and I needed to work on rotating it, so that the top of the pelvis tilted forward (reversing the process of it rolling under me).

After showing me how to tilt my pelvis and perform a mini-squat exercise (see Appendix C) to help reinforce this position, I soon felt the solid feel of my foot on the floor. The twinge in my knee also disappeared. The realization that my knee pain is due to my unconscious poor body alignment (in this case, my pelvis rolling under me caused by years of slouching) was illuminating. It was likely that my poor pelvic posture had been a major contributor to my knee injury, and poor balance in general. It taught me that we tend to do things that cause the thing we want to avoid.

I soon discovered that the pelvis rolling under is a common occurrence as we age, and probably a major reason elderly people lose their balance and fall backwards. With the pelvis rolled under, the hips to open up, and the person walks in a duck foot manner (the toes pointing outwards). This results in further slouching, causing the body's center of mass to move back, creating an unsteady gait, with heavier heel strike. It's this heavy heel strike that leads to slips, and sudden backwards falls. When this occurs in the elderly, it often results in a broken hip, which can have fatal consequences.

I further concentrated on improving my hip position in two other activities which I do daily, which are; sitting and picking up things off the floor. When I sat I made sure I pushed my rear into the seat this made me tilt my hip forward in my chair and I immediately felt my back straighten up. Stephen told me that most chairs are designed for people who are 6 feet and taller having longer upper thigh length than me. Such chairs made people with shorter thigh length not able to fit fully back into the chair causing slouching that results in hips rolling under. For such chairs I place a pillow behind me so that my upright back can rest on it and I can push my rear into the pillow preventing the urge to slouch in the chair.

The second area of activity I do that is highly hip position related is properly bending down to pick up items was taught to me by Stephen. He prescribed before you bend down take the hand that is not reaching for the item and make a karate chop hand with it and with the striking side of the hand (the little finger side) place it along the groin crease formed where upper thigh femur head and the hip socket join. As you bend down push the karate chop hand into the forming valley helping the top of the hip to tilt forward. Your rear will at the same time push out and up. You will find that several benefits in doing this beside developing good posture habit in picking items off the floor but less stress on the back, the hip, the knees and legs.

I modified Stephen's way to pick up items but still use his principles and incorporate them in both my upper body positioning as well as my hips. Before bending down cross your left hand over the right hand if you are right handed or your right hand over your left hand if you are left handed. As you bend, allow the hands to turn palm forward as you release the hand cross over and run the back of your hands over your knees (Right back of hand over the right knee, and the left back of hand over the left knee) as you reach for the item you are going to pick up. As you straighten, keep the free hand palms up.

Comment Dr. Yanuck: A major difference between my approach and Sam's comes down to muscle suppleness. My muscles lack adequate suppleness, so to achieve many of these biomechanical postures. As a result I have to continually challenge my crippled muscles (usually through physical activity) to illuminate that there is a better way biomechanically, so that those muscles will integrate that information, activate those muscles so to be amenable to healing, and I can apply techniques like ischemic compression or sequential stimulation to release spasms in them, and regain function. It is in this way that my biomechanics improve. It is a slow, gentle, gradual process, because I am so out of alignment; as a result, I can't achieve vast, sweeping changes at once, as the two sides of my body have been out of balance for so long, as to have created dysfunctional compensatory changes that have endured almost a lifetime. Hence, it requires minute changes between both side, so to undue these compensatory changes, and achieve balance.

This process has been ongoing for years. Nevertheless, I can say – definitively – that every day that I go out and physically challenge myself – on skates or skies or dancing or walking or performing these biomechanical exercises – I get better. Often, the very act of attempting Sam's recommended biomechanical approaches is enough to initiate the neuromuscular re-education process, so to trigger my crippled muscles to be amenable to healing.

And I like that. I like getting better. I marvel that I get better every day. I revel in it.

7 FOOT-HIP CONNECTION

Foot stability is directly linked to hip position. When I tilt my hip forward, the rest of my body matriculates to a very stable stance. I feel my upper legs strengthen medially, my feet firmly on the floor. Using the solid feel of my feet, I can gauge the hip tilt to afford me optimal balance.

The wonderful aspect of hip tilt is the lack of stress on the knee. Using this connection (having the feel of a firm stable foot plant) I was able to start changing the pattern of my walking to strong, stable strides.

This short section is very meaningful to me... Because I have so little foot stability – And the reason is because I was struck by that car when I was little, and the consequent damage to the muscles of my left hip, left it so I couldn't engage my left foot the way Sam describes.

So, once again, an understanding of biomechanics is great – but you also need working muscles so to be able to perform them.

At the very moment of this writing, I'm using the sequential stimulator to awaken and recover function in the muscles of my left hip, so to be able to engage this foot-hip connection...

8 ENGAGING BODY ALIGNMENT IN STRENGTHENING THE UPPER BODY ISOMETRIC TRICEPS PRESS

This exercise by Stephen Tarmibuchi utilizes body alignment to enhance the recruitment of the muscles of the triceps, shoulders, chest and back. What I like about this exercise is it helps my upper body posture especially my back.

It is an exercise that requires most of the body to be properly aligned between your feet, hands and head...

9 COMPENSATION

Muscle compensation occurs with poor alignment (i.e., engagement of inappropriate muscles to compensate for poor bio-mechanics and leverage). This compensation allows for temporary high performance, but with continued, repetitive use (especially at a high-performance level) will eventually strain the musculo-skeletal system, leading to chronic injury. Usually, the high performing athlete will realize they are having difficulty in further improvements and seek out appropriate professional coaching to define the bad habit before permanent damage occurs. However, for most of us, having the luxury of a good coach is not possible, and this is why it is critical that we develop the sensitivity of Bio-sensing to help guide us away from muscle compensation and towards proper musculo-skeletal alignment.

Comment, Dr. Yanuck: Another very insightful short section from Sam's rendering of biomechanics and healing. To rebuild a body after trauma, you likely have to overcome many compensatory processes that have been installed following an old and unreconciled injury. This is often a long and slow process, because you have to balance and equilibrate both sides of the body (back-and-forth) as you go. Such is the nature of attending the unfortunate sequelae of compensation.

10 REFERRED PAIN

A shoulder injury that occurred playing football in my freshman year of high school (and that I reinjured in a wrestling match in my sophomore year) limited the range of motion in my shoulder. Believing that I must have permanently damaged the shoulder, I basically lived with the dull ache until I was 55 years old.

But when I injured my knee and Stephen was caring for me, I asked him to examine my shoulder. Stephen said the shoulder was okay, and the pain was coming from a misalignment in my spine. After he worked on my back, the pain in my shoulder disappeared and has not reoccurred since (which has been over 10 years now). I had been living in pain, believing for over 30 years that I had a severe shoulder injury, and all along it was just a kink in my back.

This for me was a pivotal experience in understanding referred pain - that the source and cause of pain can come from distant, unrelated locations. The two surprising things were: 1. How long such an anomaly (i.e., kinked vertebrae) could last, and; 2. How easily and quickly the pain disappeared by correcting the misalignment.

Comment, Dr. Yanuck: And I would add: 3. How easily and quickly the source of the pain can be relieved and ameliorated when the correct source of pain is located, treated and reconciled. As stated elsewhere in this text, pain is trying to tell you something, and making the assumption that you're just going to have live with chronic pain for the rest of your life is often not only limiting but potentially wrong. Mostly, when it comes to soft tissue injury, the resulting physical limitations can be regained.

11 BACK TO BASICS FOR HIGHER PERFORMANCE

I frequently go back to basics, focusing on body alignment and how it affects stability and sure footedness. While rehabbing my knee, I found that when my footing was solid in its interface between the bottom of the foot and the ground, my knees also felt fine. This is in line with proper skeletal alignment, so that proper pelvic tilt (with hands palm up and forward, and my feet pointing straight or slightly inward) provides greater body stability. From this powerful position I can move into more complicated stances required for whatever performance maneuver I am trying to achieve. An example of strength leverage related to appropriate muscular-skeletal frame alignment is basketball: Forming an appropriate fist prior to shooting can afford stable body alignment, allowing not only powerful muscle recruitment, but a solid body foundation for the arms and hands to make the shot. Knowing how to align the muscular-skeletal frame creates this neutral alignment allowing the body to easily change and quickly flow in motion maintaining the body's stability for further reactive movements. Creating this dynamic bio-mechanics of cascading leverage in the muscular-skeletal alignment not only allows for the greatest power capable by the body but keeps the body in a stable balance throughout the entire movement. This is critical for minimizing injury and for allowing the chance for the body to heal as it puts minimal demand on any previously injured area.

Before I understood this, there were many times I was lured into a false sense of security that I was doing things properly; I was able to do remarkable athletic movements, only to lose them later with an accompanying injury and pain associated with a joint and/or ligaments, tendon and muscle. Muscle compensation fooled me into thinking I was doing things correctly.

Fortunately, none of this was irreversible; after proper realignment and correcting my body structure alignment, I have been able to recover if not 100%, then, at least, most functional performance.

.

12 SET-UP BEFORE I START-UP

As a continuation of getting back to basics in order to perform better, I want to mention a ritual I now do before stepping onto the roller rink. I pause right before the opening to the roller skate rink floor, and (sometimes to the dismay of the skaters behind me) I perform the following bio-mechanical set up.

1. With feet straight or slightly toe-in and arms hung down by my side with palms forward I place my left hand (the weaker hand) over my right hand then release it and allow them to swing back to my side.

2. Lifting the shoulders and rolling them back and down ending with the elbows flexed and forward in front of the rib cage.

3. The hands are palms up and the wrists slightly flexed. My head should be up looking straight ahead.

4. I then push out my rear causing just the top of my pelvis to tilt forward. I can feel my lower rear come up and the front lower part of the pelvis rotate back and slightly up. My upper body remains upward and not bent forward. My pelvis is now tilted forward at the top crest.

5. Flexing my knees just a bit I sink down and relax my body.

6. I take a deep breath in and release it as I step onto the rink and the first thing I notice is how firm the bottom of the foot is in the boot and the solid grip of wheels to the floor. I push off and begin the joy of skating.

Body preparation like this (which I call getting the body aligned in a neutral balanced stance) can be and should be done prior to any physical activity to provide a strong and safer athletic start.

13 CRAMPS, TIGHT MUSCLES AND TRIGGER POINTS

There are big differences between cramps and tight muscles, mostly related to their reasons for happening. Cramps are preludes to increase muscle coordination, and tight muscles are at first protective mechanisms. Later, tight muscles are the cause of referred pain; still later, they become an element of chronic injury (called trigger points). Release of trigger points causes the tight muscles to relax and go into a more normal state of contraction and extension. Self-release is possible but usually requires attention and appropriate action. If the muscles remain contracted, it pulls the body out of alignment, creating pain and injury along the weakest point in the chain, and then eventually other points throughout its entire length, and then throughout the entire body.

Stephen located and released these trigger points until I was able to make the movements correctly as well as build-up the appropriate muscle capacity, so not to stress and strain those muscles. Working with Dr Michael Yanuck M.D. I believe there may be a relationship between the release of trigger points and other forms of illness. Stresses that impinge the body may be detected by Bioenergy and possibly resolved. Just the act of pinpointing and sensing that area of the body subconsciously focuses our body's attention to act there. I like to think of bioenergy as a heat-seeking missile guidance system locating the trouble spot.

Trauma (at times when it happens) can cause the body to be confused. The body has a set of sequences for what it should do for most injuries, but for some abnormalities, it may have a hard time figuring out how to begin the healing process, and where to begin?

This may be part of the reason why sources of referred pain (such as trigger points) can remain for long periods, and result in issues which don't feel related. Bioenergy may help in determining the starting point for healing to begin.

Getting into the flow.

As I improved in my physical abilities I noticed that I would still strain different muscle groups. This I took as a sign that my body was slowly evolving in different movement patterns, engaging different muscles, but causing them to cramp. Ultimately, I realized I was so weak that performing more intricate coordinated athletic maneuvers was engaging un-trained and un-prepared muscles, resulting in muscle fatigue, creating poor technique and body compensation, and, done enough times, leading to the development of bad movement habits.

As I focused on posture training to arrive at neutral alignment, I slowly began to strengthen my body, so to take on the demanding maneuvers I desired. Reaching a stable, neutral posture was critical to rebuild my body, and obtain a threshold level for consistent performance with ease (and without further injury). Reaching that threshold allowed me to be in a neutral position naturally, and making it dynamic, which, in turn, allowed for flow into other different neutral positions, and continued improvements in stability and strength. Obtaining this threshold required persistence. Paramount to this effort were short, frequent practices; consistence in performing appropriate techniques; and patience guided by sensing how the body felt till eventually achieving my performance goals. This bio-sensing of the body was my internal mentor in making sure I was doing things biomechanically correctly.

Comment, Dr. Yanuck: It's interesting to me that in this small section, I see how different Sam's condition is from mine; whereas his condition (marked by sudden testosterone deficiency as a matter of hypothalamic injury) left the muscles weak, so to require better body mechanics to facilitate flow (as he was without the testosterone to power through things), my condition is a matter of muscles crippled so to literally need to be brought "back to life" (via trigger point release through methods like ischemic compression and electrostimulation) if I was to have any chance of realizing this flow. Only today (at the time of this writing) I was at The Rink, and finding that my inability to engage muscles of my lateral quadriceps was disrupting my ability to "flow" as I skated. Then, after a quick nap at home, I found those very muscles were signaling that they were ready and amenable to healing.

14 INTRA-BIOENERGY SENSING

It would be the ultimate (as well as wonderful) to always have at my fingertips the services of Dr. Yanuck to do bioenergy on me – not only after an injury, but as a preventative measure at the early onset of trouble. What I came up with was the next best thing was to have an early detection system I like to call Intra-Bioenergy sensing or BioSense. Acquiring the skill of BioSense would help us prevent our bodies from developing major problems. Because this is not a common approach in today's thinking, it is left up to us develop our body's awareness (or our personal bioenergy); it's up to us to become more sensitive to feeling and sensing what needs adjustment in our posture. My advantage to developing my own 'inner' bioenergy is that I had Dr. Yanuck to teach me to first sense it in others. I found that this gave me the capability to look for it in myself. Others who are capable of teaching bioenergy can be a great aid to help develop a sensitivity of bioenergy in ourselves, so we can improve in our posture and performance capabilities, not to mention possibly preventing future injuries.

15 A KEY CONCEPT

I adapted the concept that the body is a whole unit – a coordinated, connected, integrated system that relies on linking all parts to properly function with coordination, flexibility, strength, power, stability, effortlessness and harmony. While working on a specific area of the body, it is important to involve the body as a whole in the process for development and mending.

Comment: Around the time that Sam crafted this section, he gave me the greatest present ever for my birthday – He met me at Lake Tahoe and spent the day skiing with me. It was great – His skiing was nothing less than magical. To watch him ski was to behold a Ski Sensei, effortlessly gliding along the snow at breathtaking speeds that left me in the dust (or should I say, snow spray!). He insisted that he just wanted to spend a day with some snow under his feet; but he instructed me at every turn. I learned so much; however, the point made in this little passage was most significant – skiing with "coordination, flexibility, strength, power, stability, effortlessness and harmony." Before Sam's instruction, I'd been making turns while skiing with every part of my body; Sam taught me that balance of the body as a whole was needed, so to keep the body engaged, and prepared for anything and everything that comes next.

16 AGE AS A COLLECTION OF BAD HABITS: A FORCE THAT AGES

For me, the 'fountain of youth' I seek is the ability to mentally and physically keep improving in the activities I love. It is a simple goal, but a task that requires constant attention. Nevertheless, by striving for this, all else seems to fall in place: looking good, being good-natured, feeling joyous, adventurous, etc...

Like Newton's first law of physics: To change the direction created by a force (in this case, bad habits), a greater force needs to be applied. Because the force of the bad habits we've manifested into poor body posture has so much momentum, I read somewhere that it may takes seven times the energy and work to change it into a good habit.

And why are bad habits are so hard to change? Because the physical change caused by habitual bad posture causes other systems around it to change – just like a geographic change can cause change in climate, flora and fauna. Hence, accommodation by other systems of the body must also be overcome.

Getting back to 'fountain of youth', I had to first identify the bad habits that limited me, and then devise a plan to reverse them and install the needed good ones. My physical goal was to be a very good skier and snowboarder, as well as advance at other riding sports. My mental goal was to think and solve problems like I had in my scientific past, and apply those solutions not only to my health, but to life issues, too.

Basically, what I am saying is that when it comes to living longer, performing and doing things inefficiently (with poor bio-mechanics, alignment and posture) reinforces the bad habits which promote injuries and weakness, slow us down and eventually result in the symptoms of old age. In such a state, new injuries easily occur, as well as making it hard for the body to heal and mend. Most detrimental is when it reaches a state that we are unable to improve our abilities. Therefore, much of my journey to rebuild my body was overcoming these bad habits and replacing them with good ones that established better posture and allowed me to perform the activities I wanted to achieve.

17 WHY SKATING?

Despite improving in my skills of skiing and snowboarding, I felt an important ingredient in recovering my physical youth was lacking. More than improving my technique, I needed to be more youthful in the execution of riding sports. But who would teach me this skill?

Then it hit me like a brick falling from the heavens above: This missing vital component could be attained by learning from children by following them in their developing of riding skills.

Considering it scientifically, I decided I needed a relatively large sample population doing the same sport, as I observed how they attained success, and how they approached trying to develop their skills to do more complex riding movements. It dawned on me that the roller skating rink was the ideal place for these observation: Kids falling when attempting even the simplest skating movements, and working through it with great determination with lots of trial and error. The distribution curve was huge as I watched and rolled around the rink. I saw pretty much every attempt just to stay up and then push off to move. Older youths having the basic fundamentals of skating worked on the bit more complex moves. These moves appeared quite difficult. Attempting them myself, I realized it was my lack of relaxing that prevented me from being more agile and able to rebalance quickly (as these moves required staying over my skates in less tolerant postures). I overcame this by breaking down the movements (with the help of holding onto the back of a sofa coach in my living room through many hours of practice).

From my 'laboratory' observations at the roller rink, I discovered several things that I needed to develop: 1. The feel of communication from my feet, so that I could react from their sensors, and develop muscles unused for several decades; 2. Turning my brain off, so to stop thinking what I should do, and feel the pressure from the bottom of my feet, and throughout the kinetic body chain, and react appropriately (which I determined by studying skating technique); and 3. Smooth, effortless and timely repositioning of my body for constant dynamic changes to balance the process of moving. All of this was not easy, and what took these children achieved within a few days to weeks took me several months of methodical training and body development to be able to do only crudely. For more complex moves it would be a couple of years till it became natural to me.

But it turned out I had some advantages over my young cohorts: One – My skiing and snowboarding skills. I discovered that skating is a combination of different cross sports that combine walking, surfing and skiing. On movements that were more ski or surf-like, I had an easier time adapting than the young skaters. Another important skill I had was Judo; I was not afraid to fall, dissipating the impact, and rolling out.

Still, it is amazing to see the young skaters at times escape from falling due to their keen ability to adjust their balance. Physically, they are more stable over their feet, and typically having too much fun than to consider the possibility of bodily damage from a fall.

I wondered if I could develop such automatic behavior? The course of action I choose was relaxing, especially at my feet. Raising my toes when I skated allowed my ankles to be more flexible and adjust sooner. Although this training was accompanied by a lot of night time cramping in my legs, it built up my lower leg muscles.

Finally, breaking down the movement to feel as much as I could, I arrived at an understanding of body positions that provided the best stability and neutral alignments to allow for quick, appropriate reactions.

One further note – In observing the children, I saw two distinct groups: One group that improved quickly by discovering a technique that worked effortlessly; the other muscled their movements, and if they were able to make the move, did it in a less smooth, and more robotic manner. Regarding this latter group, since they felt they had accomplished the move (though not cleanly), they were satisfied and engrained this method as a habit (though one that minimized their ability to take on other technical moves). This latter group had good skaters, but had a lower ceiling for becoming better; while the members of the first group were able to establish good habits and techniques that allowed them to take on more difficult moves. In effect, my observations of the two groups demonstrated the long-term effects of proper and improper foundations: start with good technique, and fuller potential and broader abilities followed; establish poor technique, and there the potential for improvement and expansion was considerably diminished, as well as lending to creating poor alignment and later to poor posture.

Reflecting on my youth, I considered all the times my approach was like the kids in the second group, and what might have been had I a caring, knowledgeable coach who intervened when he noted improper technique, and taught me appropriately; I may have avoided many of the injuries I incurred, and my life have been quite different. As Marlon Brando said in the film *On the Water Front,* "I coulda been a contender."

But perhaps in not having received the coaching to become a world class athlete, I learned for myself how to coach others, studied how to get the body better, worked out smarter biomechanical practices, and hopefully the information presented here will help others recover from injury, rebound from setbacks, get beyond uncertainties, and assure that they are not alone in rebuilding their bodies.

18 MOVE FROM A POSITION OF STRENGTH TO CREATE A POWERFUL ACTION

To position and engage the body for optimally stable biomechanical advantage for dynamic neutral alignment that allows for a solid but flowing dynamic balance (as well as a rapidly explosive, efficiently smooth, powerful leveraged actions) apply the following steps:

Point 1. The Pelvis first needs to be in place to establish the foundation that the rest of the body depends on. Initiating a movement, slightly tilted the pelvis forward. You should feel your feet solidly planted on the ground. A good exercise to do is the pelvic squat (see Appendix C). This provides the measure of tilt required.

Point 2. Balance and align the body. We all have a favorite side. If you are right handed, then the right side becomes dominantly stronger and more coordinated. As we age this unevenness becomes more pronounced - not from getting older, but from greater repetitive use and actions. We become very skilled at making ourselves imbalanced with a body structure that is skewed and twisted. This can be the source of all kinds of maladies and injuries, from backaches to pinched nerves to poor circulation. From the point of athletic ability, it can be the major issues affecting agility, precision, range of motion, stability, strength of movements, and the list goes on...

Two noticeable points of the body that influence our athletic ability are the shoulders and pelvis. Usually due to the nature of being stronger on one side, the muscle-skeletal system reacts by building up that side more. If you look carefully at these two areas (the shoulder and pelvis) you find that if you are right sided that the right shoulder protrudes forward slightly more than the left, and to balance this off, set the hips left, protruding more forward than the right side. As a result, the body looks twisted like a licorice swizzle (referred to by chiropractors as "twisted butt syndrome"). This twisting body alignment weakens the bio-mechanics of the body, producing a less stable body with less powerful actions. One can temporarily counter this by just crossing the weaker side arm over the stronger arm before doing an action such as running. This will reset the body position to a neutral alignment before you perform the action; eliminating the body to work from a twisted less stable body. (see Appendix B)

Point 3. Just a small degree of angle change in the core body can affect large change in parts of the body furthest from the core. The "core" comprises the parts of your trunk that help stabilize you to resist forces of gravity and allow you to effectively operate the rest of your body. Surprisingly, despite its importance, the core can be easily displaced as a result of injury, with loss of leverage strength. And in this scenario, those parts of the body furthest from the core (the hands and feet) can actually contribute to this instability.

In this case, correcting misalignments in the core is critical. Also important is making sure that the feet and hands are not imposing instability to the structure of the body frame. The hands are the critical here, and Stephen Tamaribuchi's invention of the e3 grips or e3 gloves is a great way to assist in easily positioning the hand structure into a place the provides strong influence on body alignment and muscle recruitment. This flies in the face of trying to establish what people say about the importance of the body's core strength; however, the hands and feet can help tone the core body to align itself.

Of note, the Cub Scout hand sign helps body alignment and stability. This sign comes close to mimicking the hand position formed by the e3 grips. Forming this sign with a free hand allows the action hand and arm to be more powerful and the rest of the body more stable. I use this hand form when I do not have the e3 grips or gloves available while performing various activities.

Point 4. Consider first body parts farthest out from your core. We spoke about the hand in point 3. Now the next anatomical part is the wrist. The wrist can provide the best influence on body leverage when they are slightly flexed; your elbows best when they are closer to the body or angled close to the body; your shoulders are rounded up and back, so they are set firmly into the sockets.

From your feet start with your toes. Keep them relaxed (or slightly raised) so you can feel a little more pushed down on the balls of your feet. You will also feel your ankles more relaxed and easy to flex. The next is the foot position: Is it abducted out (in what is commonly referred to as 'duck feet' with toes angled out), straight, or toed in (also referred to as 'pigeon toed')? Straight and pigeon toed produces a stronger leverage and stronger core. Duck feet (toes point out) opens up the hip causing the pelvic to roll under and weaken the core.

Point 5. Technique development. This is mostly specific to what you want to achieve, whether it be basketball, soccer, swimming, martial arts, skiing, snowboarding, skating, surfing, volleyball, whatever requires coordinated body movements. However, there are some basic technical skills that are common to almost all these endeavors:

When moving, go from the most stable point of strength: When reaching out with your hand forward, push out with your arms from the elbows. When changing direction while walking or running, steer your feet with your heel pointing in the opposite direction. When shifting from side-to-side, turn from your hips. This can also be greatly augmented by turning your leading hand palms up (Point 3).

The closer your action point of reference to the core, the more powerful the strength of muscle leverage and recruitment.

Point 6. Practice these things as often as possible to create good body habits. Once they become natural to you, they are easily called upon for athletic activities.

19 DAILY COMMON PRACTICES THAT CREATES GOOD NATURAL HABITS AND HEALTH

I do things every day to counter my resistant bad habits of poor posture.

Sit and stand properly: Do this every time you sit and stand-up Stand to realign yourself

Picking up items off the floor: 1. Before bending down cross your left hand over the right hand if you are right handed or your right hand over your left hand if you are left handed. As you bend down allow the hands to turn palm forward as you release the hand cross over and run the back of your hands over your knees (Right back of hand over the right knee and the left back of hand over the left knee) as you reach for the item you are going to pick up. As you straighten up keep the free hand palms up. 2. An alternate way is before you bend down take the hand that is not reaching for the item and make a karate chop hand with it, and with the striking side of the hand (the little finger side) place it along the groin crease formed where upper thigh femur head and the hip socket join. As you bend down push the karate chop hand into the forming valley helping the top of the hip to tilt forward. Your rear will at the same time push out and up. You will find several benefits to doing, including developing good postural habit in picking items off the floor, with less stress on the back, hips, knees and legs.

Open a door with a stable stance
Shake hands firmly
Walking properly: Do this every time you take a step
Holding handles that minimizes injury

Flexing on one leg; do this while brushing your teeth.

20 DEALING WITH YOUR CONDITION

Know your limits and work within them and their boundaries. You may be pleasantly surprise that you can step over those boundaries one day.

Focus on what is important to achieve and do not worry about things presently beyond your grasp. Narrow it down so you can concentrate at being the best you can be.

Always keep things simple when seeking answers. Usually the simplest answers are the most correct.

In general, the only one you can truly rely on is yourself. At times you might be disappointed, but don't be angry if you do not fulfill things you thought you would or should do. Being disappointed is natural.

If you can understand why you did not reach your goals that time, you will be wiser the next time you approach with them. The same goes for others. Life is not worth being upset with yourself or others. Cherish the times when you and others come through.

Accept bad outcomes because they happen. Do damage control to reduce risk, but do not completely refrain from challenging your limits first. At times, take a loss and then look at ways to move beyond it.

Many will say why do you push yourself and especially at your age. I tell them because I can. I cannot explain what actually drives me, but I love the saying "Do what you love and everything else just falls in place" and I will add "until it can't and then it's time to look for something else to love," but if I am right about rebuilding myself then that will be a very long ways off!

Years ago I had a dream in which I envisioned a time in the future when people acquired the ability to convert matter into energy, and used it to heal. When I shared this dream with family members, they responded doubtful, and even I wonder if (in promoting bioenergy) I'm looking to set up a Jedi Knight school?

"I don't believe in the kinetics idea of using your mind to move things," Sam said. "But I do believe in your work with energy, because energy is emitted from the body, and if you can detect that energy, and use it to heal, then you're really able to help someone."

Sam talked about the importance of bioenergy with respect to injury.

"I think we're being injured all the time," he said, "and that's the thing that hinders us. Not only that, it hinders our ability to do things better. And it doesn't have to be hurting you, you could just be blocking your ability to do things better.

I knew both of things: The pain of the NIH injury that blocked my ability to continue my research into cancer vaccines; and the car accident that left me with dysfunctional muscles for most of my life.

"And so, if it can free that up," Sam said, "bioenergy can really do a lot for you."

I have written about Ginsburg's chick experiment in prior works. In that experiment he showed that chicks that were traumatized and then reconciled with the trauma did better in resiliency testing than chicks that had not been traumatized. It was only those traumatized chicks for which the process of reconciling trauma is interrupted that the trauma left the animal weaker.

So, yes, injury is part of life. We will keep injuring ourselves. But as long as we reconcile ourselves with those traumas, we make ourselves stronger.

Hence, injury and trauma is nothing to be afraid of. Indeed, they are to be embraced as normal parts of life.

"Right, exactly," Sam said. "As long as the injury isn't irreversible. As long as it's reversible, you can get better."

Unfortunately, some injury is irreversible. But the body/mind has the capacity to reconcile even those.

"It's like the old saying, 'What doesn't kill you, makes you stronger.' There's some truth to that.

Yes, it's a scientifically validated fact.

"It's like when I broke my wrist," Sam said, "and it's now stronger than my other wrist. You can feel the solidness of it.

"But, that's the thing – You have to have it healed. And that's what you're doing with your bioenergy. You are making it well-healed. You focus on it, and – boom – it's improved.

"And because of that, I think makes it so you can do better, because it re-programs your body to say, 'This is going to happen again, so let's make sure we heal it correctly this time.'"

Yes, bioenergy offers a technique that helps overcome injury and trauma, to the point that you can look forward to even life's unfortunate experiences, because in the end they just make you stronger.

"Yes, we do have on our side evolution," Sam concluded, "because Man could only survive if he was able to recover from accidents and mistakes – and he does. And accidents and mistakes we run into. That's just a normal part of life...

21 APPENDIX

Appendix A
Science and Slopes
Life's moguls bumped a workaholic to focus on training skiers
By Sam McManis
smcmanis@sacbee.com

Published: Sacramento Bee Sunday, Oct. 24, 2010 - 12:00 am | Living Here Sunday Page I1

A globe-hopping workaholic quits his dizzying schedule and finds a happy marriage between his youthful passion and his penchant for science. Sam Morishima now focuses on training skiers through Endless Slope.

STORY

A workaholic on yet another bender, logging crazy hours and crossing time zones and datelines with dizzying frequency, Sam Morishima awoke groggily one morning in 1999 with nary a clue as to his whereabouts.

With full consciousness, usually, came full clarity. Not this time.

Panicked, Morishima tried to calm himself with what he did know at that moment in that nondescript hotel room.

Your name is Sam. You're an American marketing executive for a biotech firm. You are 46, a husband, the father of one girl. You live in Sacramento. You travel frequently. You've been tiring easily, losing energy and gaining weight. Take a deep breath. You'll be OK ...

Still, nothing. Could be New Zealand. Could be Colombia. Or one of any number of locales on his itinerary.

He scurried to the table near the phone, rifled through hotel information, then consulted the schedule planner that ran his life. At last the answer: He was in Mexico City! It all came back to him.

Until, that is, a few weeks later when it happened again – this time in a hotel room in Taipei, Taiwan.

It was the weirdest thing, this temporary amnesia. To Morishima, it felt like that concussion he sustained once at a karate match. Or that time in his 20s, surfing off California's Central Coast when, caught in a riptide, he nearly drowned. Or that time at age 12 when he and a buddy scaled a 50-foot crevasse, and Morishima was briefly paralyzed with fear as his grasp slipped.

Looking back on such times, when he felt most alive yet most vulnerable, now turns Morishima introspective. The son of migrant farmworkers, the grandson of a man sent to World War II internment camps, Morishima was accustomed to finding success as a scientist through an iron will, an intense work ethic and zest for new experiences. But he remembers how the health crisis of his globe-hopping days made him question his very existence.

"I'd be gone for several weeks at a time, visiting five or six countries in a row," he recalled. "All the travel, the jet lag. time changes and biorhythm adjustments were deteriorating my health."

After myriad doctors and tests, it was determined that stalled signals from Morishima's hypothalamus had thrown his hormones into disarray. Experts told him about possible causes and treatments, but the professed workaholic knew what was wrong.

"Stress, definitely," he said. "There's no other thing. I quit work."

More than a decade later, the word "quit" still stings. Here was a kid who, at an age when most boys played with Tonka trucks, drove a tractor on the Santa Maria strawberry fields that his parents worked – by having someone put a block on the gas pedal. Here was a guy who, as a college student, hustled his way into resorts by taking church groups to Tahoe and finagling free lift tickets and lodging. Here was a hyper-vigilant employee whose biotech bosses had to force him *not* to come in to work seven days a week.

Men like him do not just quit. Sam did.

During a long night of existential dread in the year of his amnesia, Morishima mulled his future. His wife, May, was working only part time, and the family needed to save for daughter Sondra's college. But his health and spirits were low. "I need to do something physical," he thought. "It's the only way I'll survive."

Finally, near dawn, an epiphany.

"Suddenly, it hit me," he said. "Skiing."

Sophisticated treadmill

In a glorified storage shed behind the mighty Mighty Kong Cafe in Sacramento's Oak Park neighborhood, Morishima fiddled with the contraption that's been his main source of income – and the object of his obsession – for the past decade.

He calls it the Endless Slope. It's the centerpiece of his personal training business, SnoZone, which has locations in Sacramento and San Francisco, Essentially, the device is a treadmill for skiers and snowboarders to hone their craft. But comparing this sophisticated piece of machinery to a simple health-club roller would be like calling the space shuttle a turboprop.

The Endless Slope is the nexus of Morishima's new life, a happy marriage of his youthful passion for skiing and his scientist's penchant for knowing how things – motorized ski decks to human bodies – work.

The edifice of wood, steel and hard plastic, 4 feet off the ground and at an 18 percent slope, dominates the room. The light gray synthetic carpet, serving as both skiing surface and belt for the motor, is discolored from years of use. Uneven bars, like those on a gymnastic apparatus, anchor the skier, who grasps a sliding pair of hand grips to simulate poles.

All but the most advanced skiers and boarders wear a twisting harness around the waist that connects to the back bar. A fish-eye mirror at the foot of the machine reflects the skier's form back at him or her.

The Endless Slope may look like some Rube Goldberg device, but Morishima marvels at its near-Euclidean cleanness of form and function. He and an engineer built it themselves, hewing mostly to the original 1960s plans for a similar military-designed device but adding a few flourishes.

He patted the front bar like a proud father chucking his son under the chin. "It's like a Sherman tank! Indestructible! You've got to make it so it imitates snow! Ten years to perfect it! If Leonardo da Vinci knew how to snowboard, he'd have invented one of these!"

He turned reverent, remembering when he first saw a mechanical slope. It was in a San Diego parking lot, circa 1990. He filed away his interest for another time. That time came nearly a decade later. Every day for six weeks in 1999, he studied the inner workings of other revolving ski decks.

"I have to know too much about something, overdo it," he said. "It makes me feel comfortable if I understand the structure and anatomy of things."

Morishima's 86-year-old father, Kiyoshi (nicknamed Jack), recalled the time he bought Sam his first car, as payment for his years of work in the strawberry fields. It was a 1967 Chevelle Super Sport with a monster 396-cubic-inch engine. "And he took the engine apart," Jack said.

"But (my dad) also hired a mechanic to teach me how to put it back together, part by part," Sam added. "It was great. The guy taught me how to use a grocery bag for a gasket. I enjoy that kind of thing."

Skiing held a similar fascination. Even as a child, when his well-off uncle, Dr. Mitch Inouye. took him to Yosemite's Badger Pass for his first time on the slopes, Sam was drawn to the biomechanics and physics and sheer rush of the sport. Young Sam would regale friends on the farm with stories from the slopes. But he didn't leave it there.

"These are people in the fields; they'd never seen snow," he said. "My older friends with cars, I told them, 'If you drive, I'll teach you to ski.' "

Most of his fellow workers quickly lost interest in skiing, but Sam was hooked. He flirted with the idea of becoming a Tahoe ski bum, but the family's work ethic won out. Instead, he earned an academic scholarship to Santa Clara University to study biochemistry and microbiology. But he still would take church groups to Tahoe on weekends and teach them the sport.

Jack Morishima didn't know what to make of his ski-mad eldest son. "I tried to let my kids do what they wanted," he said. "But (Sam) always helped out."

Sam did not resist the strong familial pull. He left college for 2 1/2 years to help his father, who lost the farm after several poor crop years. Dad and son then worked as gardeners but saved to open their own lawn mower repair shop. Eventually, Sam was able to finish his degree.

Those ups and downs fit the family's pattern of overcoming adversity. Sam's grandfather came to the United States from Japan illegally at the turn of the 20th century. He eventually bought a melon and strawberry farm in California's Imperial Valley. The property was seized when the grandfather was sent to internment camps.

Sam's father had been in Japan visiting relatives with his mother at the time of Pearl Harbor. A teenager, Jack was drafted into the Japanese army and saw action, though he remained officially a U.S. citizen. After the war, Jack returned to California and later was drafted into the U.S. Army to serve in the Korean War.

By the time Sam was born, in 1953, the family was living in a dirt-floor house in Watsonville alongside other migrant farmworkers. But they saved enough to eventually buy farmland.

When Morishima came of age, his parents wanted a better station in life for him, and he delivered with the biotech career. Yet part of him still looked at life from a ski bum's perspective.

Morishima's wife, May, said Sam stood out in the biotech office where they met.

"Yeah, May at first thought I was the janitor," he said. Indeed, Morishima sported shoulder-length hair, wore frayed cutoffs and roller skated down the office halls to the laboratory.

"He was not the norm, to put it mildly," May said, laughing.

But the years took a toll, and the quirky chemist morphed into a paunchy, chronically stressed marketing executive – Willy Loman for the tech age. His illness convinced Morishima that he needed to find that former self.

"This," he gestured around the cramped SnoZone quarters, "is just like a laboratory. You can focus on exactly what you need to learn."

No lift ticket required

Morishima, busy now with ski season approaching, strapped in student Jon Murphy and twisted the knob. The machine hummed to life. In seconds, Murphy was schussing down the slopes – or rather, down the silicon spray-treated carpeting. Morishima leaned in, a shank of his silver-speckled black hair falling in his eyes.

"You need a little more pronation on that wedge outward," he told Murphy. "Little movements, in skiing, are more important than the big movements."

Sweat beaded, then trickled down Murphy's brow after a series of weight-transferring drills. Twenty minutes on the Endless Slope, and Murphy felt as if he'd done runs on actual slopes for a full day – absent, of course, the wintery nip in the air. Morishima tutors about 80 skiers and likes keeping numbers low to give each student attention.

"Like in a laboratory, I can notice every little change in a student," he said. "(Skiers) need to establish a path from the brain the specific muscle they need to use."

Morishima often will hop on the Endless Slope himself for a workout. He's long since shed his excess weight and now looks at least 10 years younger than 57. His health problems remain, meaning his days of daring freestyle skiing flips and snowboarding tricks are mostly behind him.

But Morishima knows where he is now and where he likes to be – skiing, both indoors and on the mountains.

"I tell you," he said, "this has saved my life."

Appendix B

Straighten the body

Secure the hip

Align the body

Recruit the appropriate muscles

Coordinate the body to work as a team by developing appropriate skills and technique for proper body movements

Practice to instill the above into daily habits of movements

Posture in:

Sitting

Standing

Walking.

Appendix C

Mini- Pelvis Squat (goal: to strengthen standing stability through improved hip position)

Taken from Stephen Tamaribuchi copy right 2010 with modification by Sam Morishima.

Modified Protocol: Exercises to improve Balance, Strength and efficiency:

2. First prepare to tilt the top of the pelvis forward by standing up right. Feet straight or slightly toe-in and arms hung down by your side holding the e3 grips* in hands with your palms forward and then lifting the shoulders and rolling them back and down ending with the elbows forward in front of the rib cage. The upper arm and elbow snug to the front side of the chest and the forearms brought up slightly above being parallel to the ground and angled out from body like curling a bar bell. The hands holding the e3 grips palms up and the wrists slightly flexed. Feels like you are flexing your biceps. The forearms are flared away from the midline of the body with elbows tucked by your sides. The flared angled out forearms are either horizontally parallel to the ground or slightly upward to 60 degrees keeping the wrists slightly flexed and the hand's palm up. Your head should be up looking straight ahead.

3. You should be standing straight up with knees locked or almost locked. In this position push out your rear causing just the top of your pelvis to tilt forward. You will feel your lower rear come up and the front lower part of the pelvis rotate back and slightly up. The upper body should remain upward and not tilt forward. Your pelvis is now tilted forward at the top crest.

4. Now relax your knees and allow them to flex down and forward just enough to unlock your knees. This will be a very small lowering of the upper body just an inch or two. You will feel a set point in the flexed knee as the body settles into this small drop. The knees should flex over the big toe, the feet pointed straight or slightly toe in. This is now your "upper referenced squat point."

5. The most important thing you should feel at this upper squat point is your feet having an improved solid and stable placement on the floor. (Stephen suggests that foot pressure should be felt on the balls of the feet especially between the first and second metatarsals and on the heels.) The weight along the foot pretty much equally distributed on the balls and the heel of both feet.

6. Inhale through the nose as you position yourself to this upper squat point.

7. From this slight knee flexed standing position (which is upper referenced squat point) squat down only 1 to 3 inches. Remember this is a mini squat and the 1 to 3-inch squat will bring down the flexed knees just slightly over the ball of the big toe. Your pelvis will rotate a bit more tilting forward as well. Important to keep the back upright and vertical. This is your "lowest squat reference point."

8. You exhale as you begin to squat down.

9. Stephen say's that you should feel no or very little pressure on the knees.

10. Hold the squat at the lowest squat reference point for 3 seconds and slowly come up and repeat the squat 4 times.

11. On the very last squat hold at the lowest squat reference point for 10 seconds and slowly come up to end.

*If no e3 grips I suggest: start off by crossing your left hand over the right hand if you are right handed or your right hand over your left hand if you are left handed then allow the arms to fall down by your side then proceed palms forward and then lifting the shoulders, etc.

Appendix D
Thoughts on Diet:
I believe Diet is important, it makes sense that toxic agents ingested is harmful if not deadly to us and lacking in certain nutrients can result in a disease state. But what is not 100% sure for me is what is a great diet or even a good diet for myself. I just do not have enough solid knowledge in this area. My approach until I can work

out this dilemma is "I try to eat in moderation." Typically, I eat what I like such as chocolates and desserts but in moderations and I eat what most would say a balanced meal for an omnivore. What I believe is what I heard from healthy individuals in my travels in countries such as Asia, Europe, Canada, Central and South America which was "when leaving a meal, you should feel a little bit hungry". It doesn't mean I follow this advice all the time, but it is at least 80% of the time.

Appendix E
Examples and approaches of others who have rebuilt themselves.
Dr. Michael Yanuck
Stephen Tamaribuchi
Anthony Sandberg
Tatsuo Okaya
Gary Ferguson...

13 EPILOGUE

Sam passed away on August 14, 2025 after a courageous battle with an incurable lung disease. For me, he was an endless source of wisdom. I was with him (at Stanford Hospital) when he got what amounted to the worst news of his life. How did he spend that evening? By offering invaluable insights to me.

I am a practitioner of Qi Gong. On that night, Sam wanted to impart his knowledge and experience in Tai Chi and Qi Gong and shared the following with me.

"When I'm doing Tai Chi and Qi Gong and feeling like I'm doing it pretty properly, it just flows," he began. "And it's amazing. I always say, at the beginning of a form, it is like slowly riding a bike uphill. I have to work at it. But once I get to a certain point, every form after that seems like they're connected.

"And then, I notice my movement speed picks up. Like it's slow at the beginning, and then once I get to a certain point it feels effortless, and all that seems to move very smoothly, and linking each movement, so it seems like one leads right into the next one, and it feels so effortless.

"And my breathing isn't hard, so it feels really good. In fact, my breathing is more in sync and it feels so comfortable.

"Oh, Mike, like I feel like a little kid, riding down a mountain road, going downhill, with my mouth open, and feeling the rush of air, and my hair flowing back, and my legs are just effortlessly peddling the bike. And it's a really neat feeling.

"In a way, I feel very, very grateful for the condition I'm in. Because if I was really healthy, there wouldn't have been any motivation to do any of this.

"In fact, if I was really healthy, I wouldn't have done Tai Chi or Qi Gong at all. As I was growing up, I always felt Tai Chi was kind of a silly thing to do. And Qi Gong was silly. I felt like, 'I don't want to do Tai Chi. I don't want to do Qi Gong. I don't have the time. I have no need for it. I'm healthy. I can do things. There wasn't any need for that.' It's only when I got this illness.

"That's why I always say, the bad things – the worst things – that have happened in my life have been my greatest teachers..."

In general, Sam was full of life. When we'd go up to the slopes, I came to so admire his skiing that it was all I wanted to do. He was kind, selfless, and a source of beauty and inspiration. Being with him on the slopes was simply magical, like beholding a 'Ski Sensei', right out of the pages of Richard Bach's Illusions. There's no one I so dearly miss.

ABOUT THE AUTHORS

Sam Morishima graduated Santa Clara University
with a degree in biochemistry and microbiology. He began
his career as a chemist, then worked for years in the biotechnology
industry, performing international sales, marketing and business
development for companies all over California, Europe, Latin
America, Asia and the Pacific Rim. Following an incapacitating
illness, he focused on healing himself and rebuilding his damaged
body. Embracing his passion for skiing, his condition stabilized
and health improved, he established a ski school
to help others by sharing his knowledge.

Michael Yanuck MD PhD is a physician-scientist
whose groundbreaking research at the National Institutes of
Health was the basis for an FDA-approved vaccine for cancer.
Following a traumatic leg injury, he trained in Bioenergy and Qi
Gong, introduced Energy Medicine techniques at the National
Center for Complementary and Integrative Health, and worked with
Qi Gong Masters who were part of the President's Executive
Committee on Alternative Medicine. For his work with Veterans,
he received the 2023 Science of Tai Chi & Qigong Award.
At the University of California-Davis, he co-led the
Long COVID-Qi Gong study, providing hope for
those with long COVID.

www.ingramcontent.com/pod-product-compliance
Lightning Source LLC
Chambersburg PA
CBHW032121280326
41933CB00009B/940